The Muscle Book

Paul Blakey

Himalayan Institute Press
Honesdale, Pennsylvania

Printed and distributed in the USA by
Himalayan Institute Press
RR 1 Box 1129
Honesdale, Pennsylvania 18431

© 1992 Bibliotek Books Ltd
19 Warwick Road
Stafford, ST17 4PD UK

9 8 7 6 5 4 3 2 1

The paper used in this publication meets the minimum requirements of American
National Standard for Information Sciences—Permanence of Paper for Printed Library
Materials, ANSI Z39.48-1984.

ISBN 0-89389-182-7

Disclaimer
The author and publisher of this material are not liable or responsible to any person
for any damage caused or alleged to be caused directly or indirectly by the information
in this book. If you are in doubt, consult a physician.

Dedication

The idea for this book germinated when I started teaching anatomy and physiology to dance students at the Merseyside Dance Centre, Liverpool, England.

It was obvious from my attempts to find suitable textbooks that most were inappropriate. What was needed was something like a car repair manual. You know the sort - it starts with a diagram of the car so you can locate the bit you want, followed by detailed information about specific parts showing how they relate to the whole.

That's what I've tried to do for you. I hope you like it.

Many thanks to Gaynor Owen, John and Mary Salisbury, and Nicky, Gemma and Saul for helping me.

And to all my teachers everywhere I say a huge thank you.

Paul Blakey

Contents

How to use this book

This is your personal body parts manual. It is about muscles - what they look like, what they are attached to, what they move, what happens when they weaken, what to watch out for to avoid injury, and some simple finger first-aid.

Apart from a few pages at the beginning and at the end, all the muscle pages have a similar format. They include most or all of the elements shown below.

The **name** of the muscle, with an explanation of the origins of the term.

A **line drawing** of the muscle

The **body language of weakness** - a description of movement difficulties which indicate problems involving the muscle.

Finger first aid diagrams showing pressure points and massage therapy to strengthen weak muscles (see also origin and insertion massage).

Movements which cause stress and strain on the muscle, under the heading **WATCH OUT!** This section aims to prevent injury by developing your awareness and understanding.

The **action** of the muscle - the movement of the body that it produces.

The **origin** of the muscle - the attachment point which does not move when the muscle contracts.

The **insertion** of the muscle - the attachment point that does move when the muscle contracts.

The muscle's **synergists** - other muscles which contribute to the action of the principal muscle.

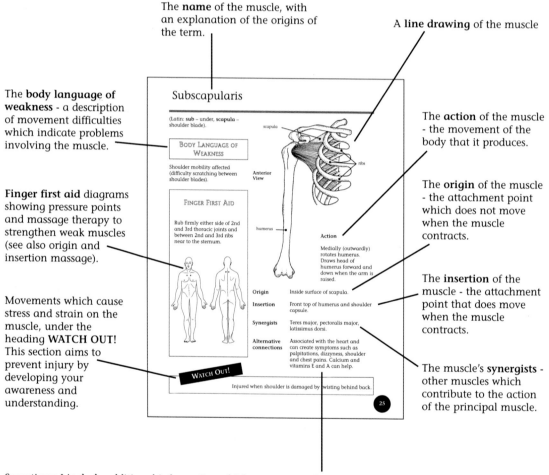

Subscapularis

(Latin: **sub** – under, **scapula** – shoulder blade).

BODY LANGUAGE OF WEAKNESS

Shoulder mobility affected (difficulty scratching between shoulder blades).

Anterior View

scapula

ribs

FINGER FIRST AID

Rub firmly either side of 2nd and 3rd thoracic joints and between 2nd and 3rd ribs near to the sternum.

humerus

Action

Medially (outwardly) rotates humerus. Draws head of humerus forward and down when the arm is raised.

Origin — Inside surface of scapula.

Insertion — Front top of humerus and shoulder capsule.

Synergists — Teres major, pectoralis major, latissimus dorsi.

Alternative connections — Associated with the heart and can create symptoms such as palpitations, dizzyness, shoulder and chest pains. Calcium and vitamins E and A can help.

WATCH OUT!

Injured when shoulder is damaged by twisting behind back.

25

Sometimes I include additional information which you may wish to consider in relation to specific body problems - for example about nutrition. This is found under the Alternative Connections heading.

On pages 6, 7, 8, and 9 you will find front and back views of the body showing the skeleton and muscles. These are reference pages which help you to see where muscles are located in relation to the whole body.

You can refer back to these from individual muscle pages, or use them as a kind of index if you know where a muscle is but not what it is called.

Anatomical terminology

I have tried to keep jargon to a minimum in this book, but some anatomical terminology is essential. This is simply because it is the most economical way of describing movement or relations of body parts to one another.

Regarding muscle actions, it is necessary to learn the following terms;

- **Flexion.** This means bending or folding. Flexor muscles generally curl the body forward into the foetal position. Toe flexors curl the toes.

- **Extension.** This means stretching out. Extensor muscles stretch the body, as in bending backwards with arms over the head.

Flexors and extensors oppose one another.

- **Rotation.** This means turning round, like a wheel. In anatomical terms it means movement around the axis of a bone.

- **Abduction.** This means taking or drawing away. In body terms it is a movement to the side by one muscle moving away from another, as in lifting a limb away from the body.

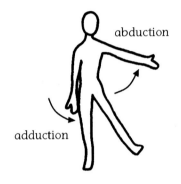

- **Adduction.** This means drawing inward. It is a sideways movement opposite to abduction, for example bringing a limb towards the centre of the body.

Adductors and abductors oppose one another.

Origin and Insertion Technique

You will come across this term frequently in the Finger First Aid sections. It is a method of stimulating or 'waking up' a weak muscle. The origin and insertion points are the places where the muscle attaches to the bone. All you have to do to stimulate the muscle is to place your fingers at these points and rub firmly across the fibres.

This technique works very well on muscles that have been strained or overworked. It stimulates the circulation and particularly the lymphatic system. It con be repeated frequently until the weakness and stiffness have gone.

Reference page 1

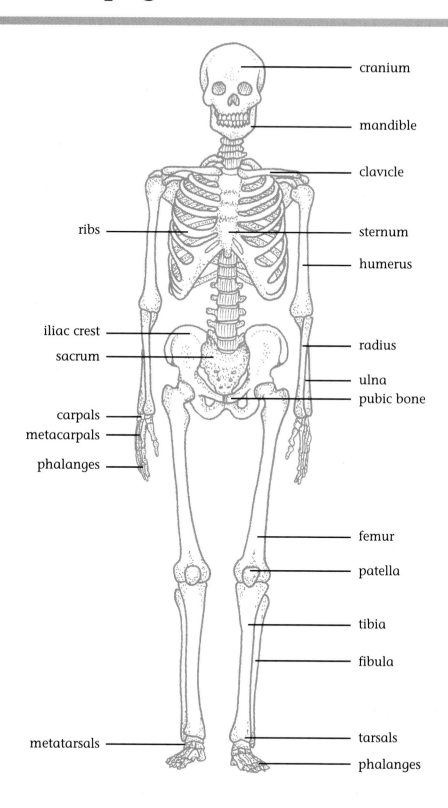

cranium

mandible

clavicle

ribs

sternum

humerus

iliac crest

sacrum

radius

ulna
pubic bone

carpals

metacarpals

phalanges

femur

patella

tibia

fibula

metatarsals

tarsals

phalanges

Reference page 2

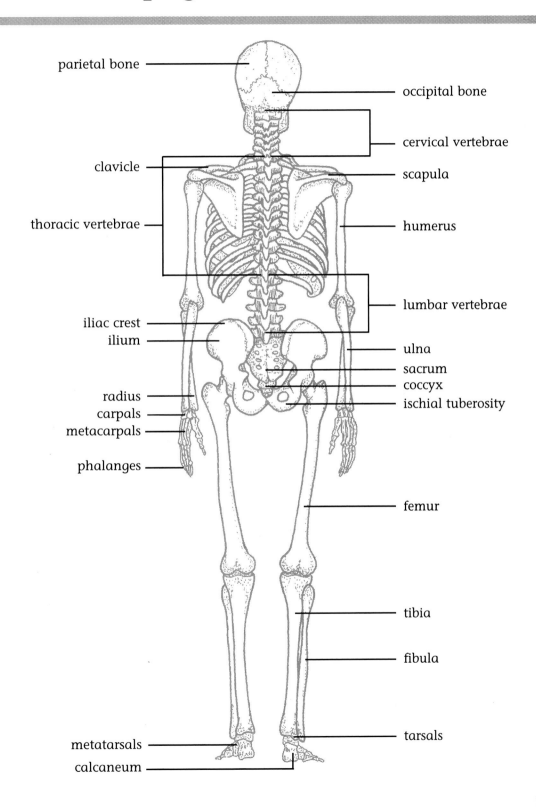

parietal bone

occipital bone

cervical vertebrae

clavicle

scapula

thoracic vertebrae

humerus

lumbar vertebrae

iliac crest

ilium

ulna

sacrum

coccyx

radius

ischial tuberosity

carpals

metacarpals

phalanges

femur

tibia

fibula

tarsals

metatarsals

calcaneum

Reference page 3

sternocleidomastoid (10)

deltoid (22)

pectoralis major (21)

biceps (14)

abdominals (45)

wrist flexors (15)

tensor fascia lata (39)

quadriceps (36)

peroneus (32)

anterior tibial (30)

subscapularis (25)

serratus anterior (19)

psoas (44)

iliacus (44)

sartorius (37)

adductors (40)

This page and the next show the muscles of the body and the pages on which more information can be found about each one.

Reference page 4

levator scapulae (13)

trapezius (16)

supraspinatus (23)

deltoid (22)

infraspinatus (27)

teres minor (26)

rhomboid (17)

teres major (24)

triceps (13)

latissimus dorsi (20)

sacrospinalis (11)

quadratus lumborum(12)

wrist extensors (15)

gluteus medius (41)

piriformis (42)

gluteus maximus (43)

gracilis (38)

hamstrings (35)

gastrocnemius (28)

soleus (29)

posterior tibial (31)

Sternocleidomastoid

Attached to the **sternum**, **clavicle** and **mastoid** bone.

Difficulty raising head from supine (lying on your back) position.

Head turns towards the weak side when lying down.

Neck extension increases, forming an 'S' curve.

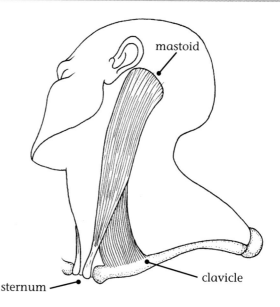

sternum · clavicle · mastoid

FINGER FIRST AID

To strengthen these muscles, rub the origin and insertion.

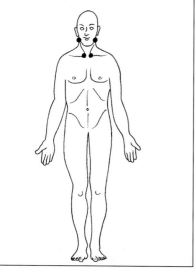

Action	Both together, flexes head. One only, rotates head and draws it towards shoulder.
Origin	Top of the sternum and first third of clavicle.
Insertion	Mastoid process of the skull, at the back of the head, behind the ears.
Synergists	Neck flexors.
Alternative connections	These muscles are also associated with the sinuses and can be affected by allergies, producing headaches and neck tension. B vitamins can help.

WATCH OUT!

Violent whiplash movements cause injury to these muscles. They play a minor role in supporting the head in relation to balance reflexes and even minor strains can upset the body's structural alignment.

Sacrospinalis

(Latin: **sacrum** - holy, **spina** - thorn).

BODY LANGUAGE OF WEAKNESS

Weakness on one side will cause a sideways bending. Both sides weak will result in a round-shouldered, slouching posture. The strong side will often stand out like a rope or cord down one side of the spine.

FINGER FIRST AID

To strengthen, press firmly with your thumbs either side, down the length of the spine. Also press firmly (but not too hard) either side of the navel.

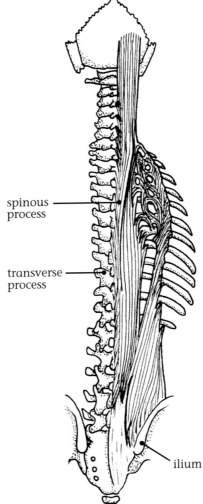

spinous process

transverse process

ilium

Action

Extension, lateral flexion and rotation of vertebral column; lateral movement of pelvis. (Bending backwards, bending sideways and twisting spine).

Origin

Separate slips of muscle arising from the sacrum, crest of the ilium, spinous processes, transverse processes and ribs.

Insertion

Into the ribs, transverse processes, spinous processes and occipital bone.

Alternative connections

Closely associated with the emotional aspects of bladder problems, (being unable to 'let go' of tension). Difficulty in eliminating the unwanted. Vitamins C and A can help.

WATCH OUT!

Avoid bending, stretching forward and lifting at the same time.

Quadratus Lumborum

(Latin: **quad** - four, **lumbar** - loin).

Weakness on one side will show as an elevation of the 12th rib and a curve in the lumbar vertebrae (leaning away from the weak side).

FINGER FIRST AID

To strengthen, massage firmly either side of L5 (fifth lumbar vertebra). Also just inside the top front edge of the iliac crest and the top half of the inside of the thigh.

12th rib

iliac crest

WATCH OUT!

Excessive side bending can injure this muscle, especially if done quickly.

Action	Lateral flexion (side bending) of lumbar vertebrae, depression of 12th rib; assistance of diaphragm in inspiration.
Origin	Top rear of iliac crest, and ilio-lumbar ligament.
Insertion	Bottom edge of 12th rib, transverse processes of the upper four lumbar vertebrae.
Synergists	Internal and external oblique abdominals, psoas major.
Alternative connections	Can often be involved when there is an intervertebral disk injury.

Triceps

(Latin: **tri** - three, **caput** - head).

BODY LANGUAGE OF WEAKNESS

Arm remains bent if you try to straighten it above the head.

FINGER FIRST AID

Rub origins and insertion (top and bottom of humerus at the back).

clavicle

humerus

scapula

Posterior View

ulna

Action	Extends (straightens) forearm.
Origin	Top rear of humerus, outer edge of scapula below joint, rear of humerus just above the elbow.
Insertion	Ulna, below elbow.
Alternative connections	The proper function of this muscle can be affected by problems involving sugar metabolism. Vitamin A can help, as can avoiding excess refined sugar.

WATCH OUT!

Falling on the hand when the arm is bent or forceful throwing can injure the triceps tendon.

Biceps

(Latin: **bi** - two, **caput** - head).

BODY LANGUAGE OF WEAKNESS

When standing the elbow is held in extension (straight).

FINGER FIRST AID

Rub origins and insertions (top and bottom of humerus at the front).

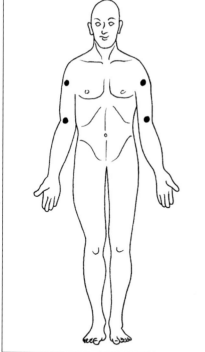

WATCH OUT!

Injury to the biceps tendon can occur when lifting or throwing heavy objects.

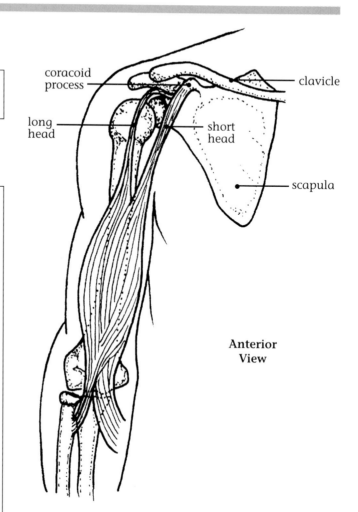

coracoid process

clavicle

long head

short head

scapula

Anterior View

Action	Flexes (bends) and supinates (turns palm upwards) the forearm. Also active when shoulder is flexed.
Origin	Short head: scapula, tip of coracoid process. Long head: top of the scapula, at the joint.
Insertion	Radius and deep fascia (connective tissue) of the forearm flexor muscles.
Alternative connections	Associated with nervous tension and insomnia.

Wrist Flexors/Wrist Extensors

Wrist benders and stretchers, and finger movers.

Inability to grip.

FINGER FIRST AID

Pain on the outside of the elbow can often be relieved by firm pressure into the origin (medial and lateral epicondyle of humerus) and belly of these muscles.

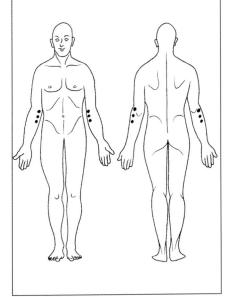

WATCH OUT!

Most injuries of the wrist involve falling onto the hand, either spraining or fracturing the joint.

Action	**Flexors** flex the wrist (palms upwards, bend wrist up towards body). **Extensors** extend the wrist (palms downwards, bend hand up towards body).
Origin	**Flexors:** medial epicondyle, (bump on the inside bottom of humerus), upper radius and ulna and interosseus membrane (membrane between the two bones). **Extensors:** lateral epicondyle, (bump on the outside bottom of humerus) and upper parts of the bones and interosseus membrane of the forearm.
Insertion	**Flexors:** carpal, metacarpal bones and phalanges. **Extensors:** carpal, metacarpal bones and distal phalanges (fingers).
Alternative connections	Tension in these muscles often means that you can't 'let go' of something in your life.

Trapezius (upper, middle and lower)

(Latin: **trapeza** - table, four sides not parallel).

FINGER FIRST AID

Midway between the shoulder and neck press firmly. Massage down either side of the spine from the neck to the bottom ribs. Pay special attention to the area between the shoulder blades and spine.

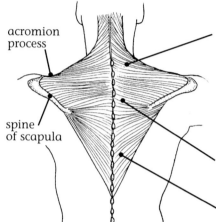

acromion process

spine of scapula

Action

Upper: adducts and rotates scapula, laterally flexes neck and head, rotates head away from the side which is contracting.
Middle: adducts and slightly elevates scapula.
Lower: rotates scapula, helps maintain spine in extension.

Origin	**Upper**: base of the skull, along spine to C7 (7th cervical joint). **Middle**: spinous processes of 1st to 5th thoracic vertebrae. **Lower**: spinous processes, 6th to 12th thoracic vertebrae.
Insertion	**Upper**: lateral third of clavicle and acromion process. **Middle**: upper border of spine of scapula. **Lower**: medial third of spine of scapula.
Synergists	**Upper**: Levator scapulae, sternocleidomastoid. **Middle**: rhomboids.
Alternative connections	The upper trapezius is associated with eye and ear problems. The middle and lower can be especially affected by infections, sore throats and fevers. Vitamins A, B and C can help.

WATCH OUT!

These muscles often become hypertonic (too tight) due to dance (particularly ballet) training, causing discomfort and restriction of mobility. Most neck and upper back stiffness in dancers is due to excess tension in this area.

Rhomboids

(Greek: **rhomb**: an equilateral parallelogram).

Complaints of aching and soreness between shoulder blades. Excessive military posture (shoulders pulled back), a sign of tension.

FINGER FIRST AID

Deep massage between shoulder blades and stretching, pressing the scapula away from the spine.

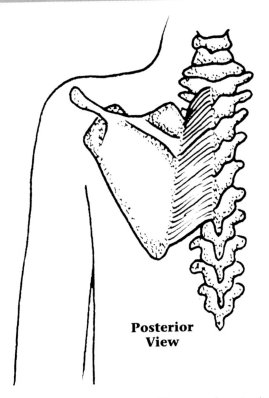

Posterior View

Action	Adducts (pulls towards spine) the scapula.
Origin	Spinous processes of the 7th cervical vertebra and the upper 5 thoracic vertebrae.
Insertion	Medial (inner) border of scapula.
Synergists	Trapezius, levator scapulae and latissimus dorsi.
Alternative connections	Associated with liver function.

WATCH OUT!

Like the trapezius, usually hypertonic (too tight).

17

Levator Scapulae

(Latin: **levator** - lifter, **scapula** - shoulder blade).

Lack of normal scapular mobility.

FINGER FIRST AID

Press firmly the belly of the teres minor muscle, also the intercostal space below the 1st rib near to the sternum (these are reflex points). Also massage origin and insertion (often the tendon of this muscle can be felt like a tight cord where it inserts into the scapula).

Posterior View

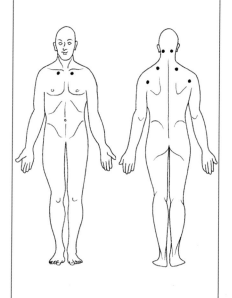

Action	In combination with trapezius, elevates and adducts scapula. When scapula fixed, flexes and slightly rotates cervical spine.
Origin	Transverse processes of four upper cervical vertebrae.
Insertion	Top of scapula closest to the spine.
Synergists	Rhomboids and trapezius.

WATCH OUT!

Usually hypertonic (too tight), affecting mobility of neck in rotation and side bending.

Serratus Anterior

(Latin: **serra** - saw, **anterior** - in front).

Difficulty pushing with arms straight out in front. Holding a weight in front will cause scapular 'winging'.

FINGER FIRST AID

Press firmly either side of the spine at the level of T3-T5 (3rd to 5th thoracic joints). Also between 3rd, 4th and 5th ribs near to the sternum.

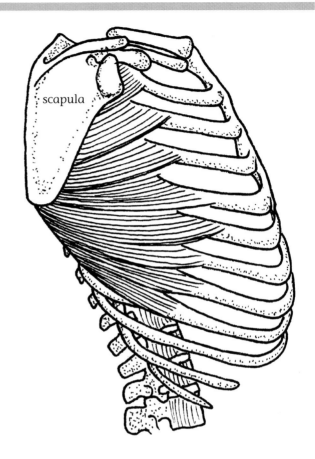

scapula

Action	Draws scapula forward against the ribs.
Origin	Outer surface of the upper 8 or 9 ribs.
Insertion	Inner surface of scapula along the medial edge nearest the spine.
Alternative connections	Can be affected by chest conditions or breathing difficulties. Vitamin C helps.

WATCH OUT!

Imbalances between serratus anterior and rhomboids or trapezius all cause tension problems in regard to shoulder mobility.

Latissimus Dorsi

(Latin: **latus** - broad, **dorsum** - back).

BODY LANGUAGE OF WEAKNESS

Uneven shoulders, higher on the weak side due to contraction of the unopposed trapezius. An inability to do climbing movements, such as chin-ups.

FINGER FIRST AID

Either side of T7-T8, use firm pressure. Also massage origin and insertion.

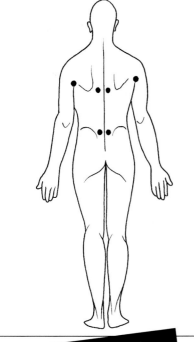

WATCH OUT!

Damage to this muscle can affect shoulder mobility.

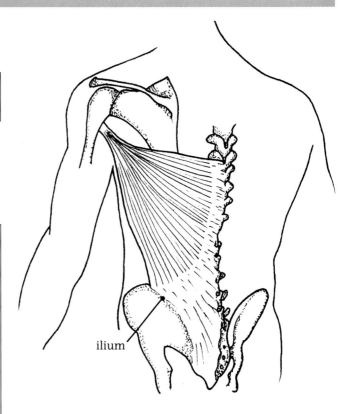

ilium

Action	Extends, adducts and rotates the humerus medially (draws the arm back and inwards towards the body).
Origin	A broad sheet of tendon originating from the spinous processes of the six lower thoracic and the five lumbar vertebrae; also the posterior crest of the ilium.
Insertion	Twists to insert into the humerus just below the shoulder.
Alternative connections	Very sensitive to problems with sugar metabolism. Can also be an indication (if chronically weak), of possible allergies and intolerance to caffeine and tobacco. Avoid excess sugar. Vitamin A helps.

Pectoralis Major (Clavicular and Sternal)

(Latin: **pectoris** - the breast).

Clavicular: difficulty moving arms across chest in a horizontal position.

Sternal: diminished ability to make quick, downward thrusting movements (like the crawl in swimming).

FINGER FIRST AID

These muscles are markedly affected by emotional stress and often a few minutes of light contact on the frontal eminences (points on the forehead, above the eyes), will do more than hours of massage. If the problem is simple physical exhaustion then rub the origin and insertion.

Anterior View

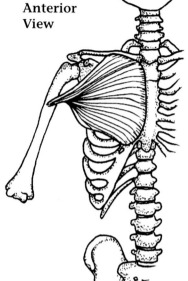

Action

Medial rotation of the humerus.
Clavicular: flexes the shoulder and horizontally adducts humerus.
Sternal: adducts humerus towards opposite iliac crest, major anterior shoulder stabiliser.

Origin

Clavicular: front surface of sternal half of the clavicle.
Sternal: sternum and adjacent parts of upper 7 ribs.

Insertion

Clavicular: top of the humerus under the front edge of the deltoid.
Sternal: same as clavicular.

Synergists

Clavicular: Biceps, sternal part of pectoralis major.
Sternal: Latissimus dorsi, subscapularis, teres major.

Alternative connections

This muscle is connected to reflexes which involve both the stomach and emotional centres in the brain. Possibility of problems with allergies. Vitamin B helps.

WATCH OUT!

The insertion of this muscle is the most likely area for injury, but usually this is limited to injuries sustained during weight training or other strength activities such as wrestling, shot putting or javelin throwing.

Deltoid

(Greek: **delta** - the fourth letter in the Greek alphabet, shaped like a triangle).

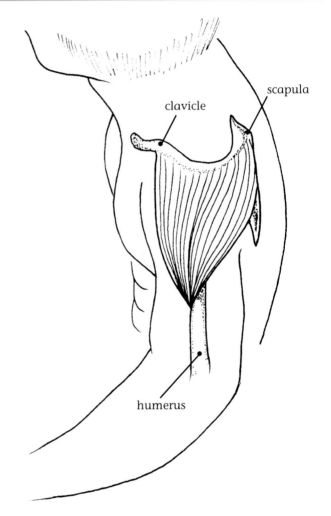

clavicle

scapula

humerus

BODY LANGUAGE OF WEAKNESS

Difficulty holding arm out to the side.

FINGER FIRST AID

Front of body, between 3rd, 4th and 5th ribs near sternum. Back of body, either side of 3rd, 4th and 5th thoracic joints. Use firm pressure.

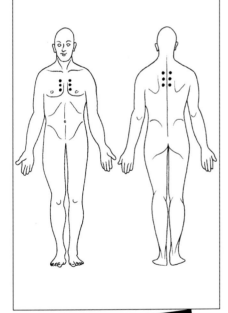

WATCH OUT!

A strong muscle, usually only injured if the shoulder joint is severely damaged.

Action	Abducts the shoulder (lifts away from the body), flexes and extends the arm.
Origin	Clavicle and spine of the scapula.
Insertion	Side of humerus.
Synergists	Supraspinatus.
Alternative connections	Lung problems such as bronchitis, pleurisy, pneumonia and flu will affect this muscle. Vitamin C helps.

Supraspinatus

(Latin: **supra** - above, spine of scapula).

BODY LANGUAGE OF WEAKNESS

Difficulty moving the arm away from the body.

FINGER FIRST AID

Rub firmly the groove between the chest and arm. Also rub under the skull where it joins the neck.

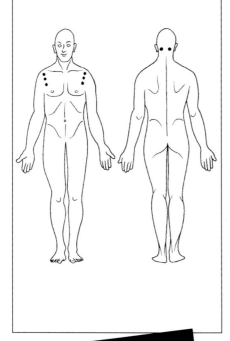

WATCH OUT!

A shoulder dislocation will damage this muscle.

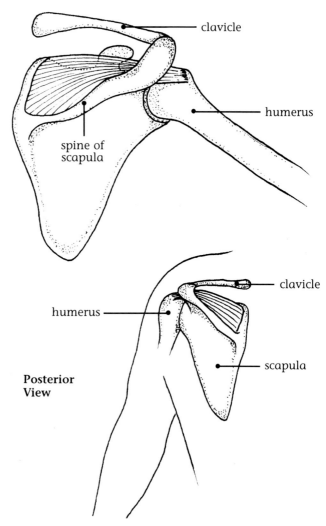

clavicle

humerus

spine of scapula

Posterior View

humerus

clavicle

scapula

Action	Abducts arm with deltoid. Holds humerus in shoulder socket.
Origin	Scapula, above the spine of the scapula.
Insertion	Top of the humerus.
Synergists	Deltoid.
Alternative connections	Intense concentration, such as driving or working at a desk, often fatigues this muscle.

23

Teres Major

(Latin: **teres** - smooth, **major** - big).

BODY LANGUAGE OF WEAKNESS

Difficulty reaching behind and drawing the elbow backwards.

FINGER FIRST AID

Rub origin and insertion. Also either side of 2nd and 3rd thoracic joints and between 2nd and 3rd ribs, 2-3 inches from the sternum.

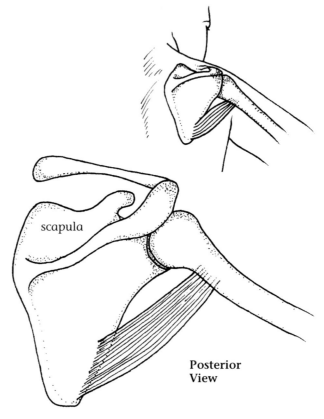

scapula

Posterior View

Action	Adducts (pulls inwards) and medially (inwardly) rotates humerus. Extends shoulder joint.
Origin	Bottom lateral edge of scapula.
Insertion	Back of humerus just below shoulder joint.

WATCH OUT!

Jerking the arm forwards sharply will damage this muscle.

Subscapularis

(Latin: **sub** - under, **scapula** - shoulder blade).

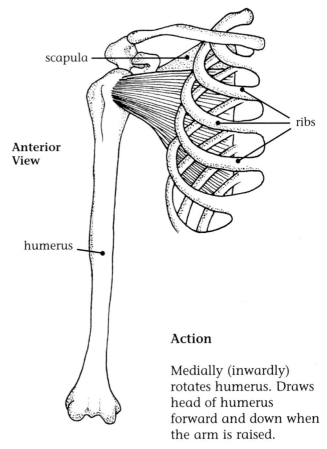

scapula

ribs

Anterior View

humerus

FINGER FIRST AID

Rub firmly either side of 2nd and 3rd thoracic joints and between 2nd and 3rd ribs near to the sternum.

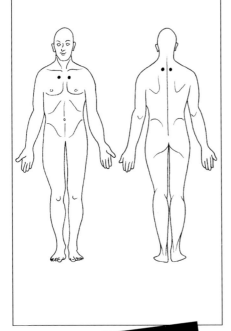

Action

Medially (inwardly) rotates humerus. Draws head of humerus forward and down when the arm is raised.

Origin	Inside surface of scapula.
Insertion	Front top of humerus and shoulder capsule.
Synergists	Teres major, pectoralis major, latissimus dorsi.
Alternative connections	Associated with the heart, and can create symptoms such as palpitations, dizziness, shoulder and chest pains. Calcium and vitamins E and A can help.

WATCH OUT!

Injured when shoulder is damaged by twisting behind back.

Teres Minor

(Latin: **teres** - smooth, **minor** - small).

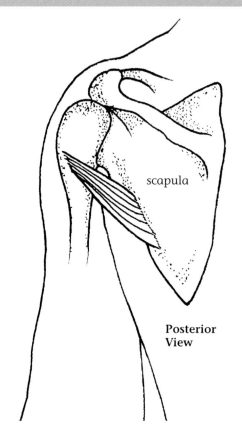

scapula

Posterior View

<table>
<tr><td>

BODY LANGUAGE OF WEAKNESS

When the hands hang down by the side, the palms will face backwards.

FINGER FIRST AID

Rub firmly either side of 2nd and 3rd thoracic joints and between 2nd and 3rd ribs near to the sternum. Also rub origin and insertion.

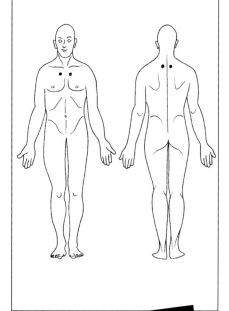

</td></tr>
</table>

Action	Laterally (outwardly) rotates humerus. Also slightly adducts and extends. Stabilises humerus in shoulder socket.
Origin	Edge of scapula closest to arm.
Insertion	Top of humerus at the back. Shoulder capsule.
Synergists	Infraspinatus.
Alternative connections	Wrist and elbow problems can develop as compensation for a weak teres minor.

WATCH OUT!

Jerking and twisting the arm will damage this muscle.

26

Infraspinatus

(Latin: **infra** - below, spine of the scapula).

Palms face backwards when arms are relaxed.

FINGER FIRST AID

Massage whole muscle.

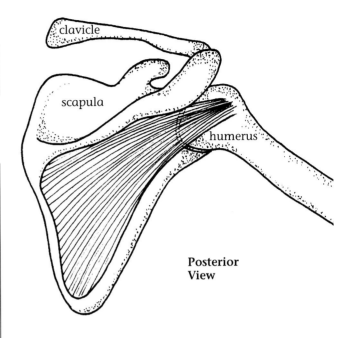

clavicle

scapula

humerus

**Posterior
View**

Action	Lateral rotation of humerus with teres minor. Stabilises head of humerus within the shoulder socket.
Origin	Middle two-thirds of scapula below spine of scapula.
Insertion	Top of humerus, shoulder joint capsule.
Synergists	Teres minor.

WATCH OUT!

One of the rotator cuff muscles. Always injured if the shoulder joint is damaged.

Gastrocnemius

(Greek: **gaster** - belly, **kneme** - leg).

Hyperextended knees.

FINGER FIRST AID

Stretch and massage whole muscle. Also press firmly 2 finger widths above and either side of the navel and either side of the 10th, 11th and 12th thoracic vertebrae.

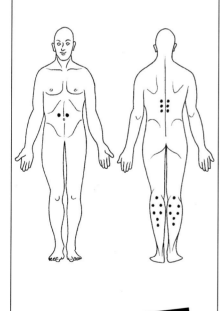

Action

Plantar flexion of foot (pointing the foot or rising onto demi-pointe).

Origin

Back of the leg, just above the knee.

Insertion

Via the Achilles tendon, into the heel bone.

Synergists

Soleus, posterior tibial, peroneus longus/brevis, flexor hallucis and digitorum longus.

Alternative connections

Emotional stress, fatigue and mild shock can affect the strength of this muscle. Vitamin C helps.

tibia

tendon

WATCH OUT!

Ruptures are common at the point where the Achilles tendon merges with the inner belly of the calf muscle. Usually caused by jumping.

Soleus

(Latin: **soles** - sole, flat).

FINGER FIRST AID

Stretch and massage whole muscle. Also press firmly two finger widths above and either side of the navel and either side of the 10th, 11th and 12th thoracic vertebrae.

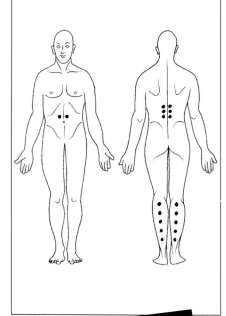

Action

Plantar flexion of foot (in isolation, rising onto demi-pointe with knees bent).

Origin

Outside back of leg, just below the knee.

Insertion

Via the Achilles tendon, into the heel bone.

Synergists

Gastrocnemius, posterior tibial, peroneus longus/brevis, flexor hallucis and digitorum longus.

Alternative connections

Emotional stress, adrenal exhaustion and shock can affect the strength of this muscle. Vitamin C helps.

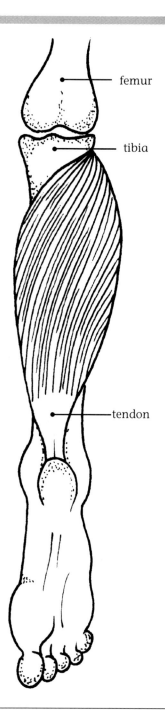

femur

tibia

tendon

WATCH OUT!

Ruptures are common at the point where the Achilles tendon merges with the inner belly of the calf muscle. Usually caused by jumping.

Anterior Tibial

(Latin: **anterior** - in front, **tibia** - shinbone, flute).

Weakness in this muscle can lead to 'rolling' inwards due to the collapsing medial longitudinal arch of the foot.

FINGER FIRST AID

Press firmly just above the pubic bone and either side of the 2nd lumbar vertebra. Also massage whole muscle.

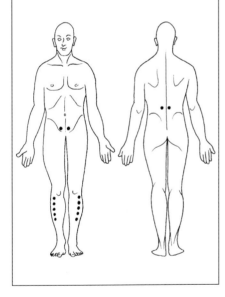

Action

Dorsiflexes (lifts up) and inverts the foot.

Origin

Outer side of tibia, just below the knee at the front.

Insertion

Inner edge of the foot, about two inches from the big toe.

Synergists

Extensor hallucis longus, extensor digitorum longus.

Alternative connections

Associated with bladder problems. Vitamin E helps.

WATCH OUT!

Often associated with 'shin splints', it is this muscle that aches from jumping on hard surfaces.

Posterior Tibial

(Latin: **posterior** - behind, **tibia** - shinbone, flute).

BODY LANGUAGE OF WEAKNESS

'Rolling' inwards and instability of ankle on pointe and demi-pointe.

FINGER FIRST AID

Reflex points - press firmly 2 inches above and 1 inch to either side of the navel. Also either side of the 11th and 12th thoracic vertebrae.

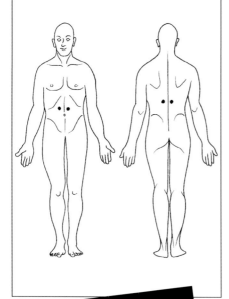

WATCH OUT!

Action

Plantar flexes and inverts the foot. (What every dancer dreads to see when pointing the foot.)

Origin

Back of the tibia and fibula, and the interosseus membrane just below the knee.

Insertion

Medial tarsal and metatarsal bones.

Synergists

Flexor hallucis longus, flexor digitorum longus, gastrocnemius, soleus.

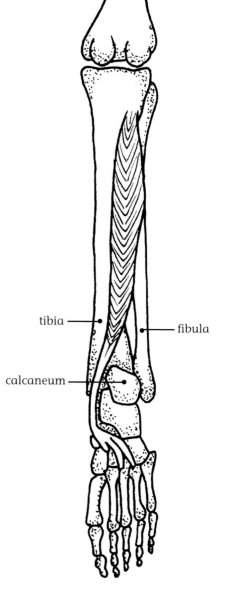

tibia

fibula

calcaneum

Turning out the feet from the ankles rather than the knees causes this muscle to stretch so that the medial longitudinal arch drops.

31

Peroneus Longus/Brevis

(Greek **perone** - fibula. Latin: longus - long, **brevis** - short).

A tendency to 'go over' onto the outside of the ankle.

Origin and insertion technique. Also massage whole muscle.

peronius longus

peronius brevis

Action	Plantar flexes (points) and everts the foot. Gives lateral (sideways) stability to the ankle.
Origin	Outer side of the leg, attached to the fibula.
Insertion	Longus: 1st metatarsal. Brevis: 5th metatarsal.
Synergists	Gastrocnemius, soleus.

Spraining this muscle by going over onto the outside of the ankle causes injury which if not treated properly can cause many problems involving the future stability of the joint.

Flexor Hallucis Longus

(Latin: **flexum**- to bend, **hallux** - big toe).

FINGER FIRST AID

Massage and stretch under side of foot by pulling the big toe towards the knee.

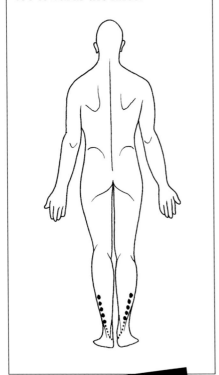

Action

Flexes big toe. Helps stabilise inside of ankle.

Origin

Lower two-thirds of the back of the fibula.

Insertion

Last phalanx of big toe.

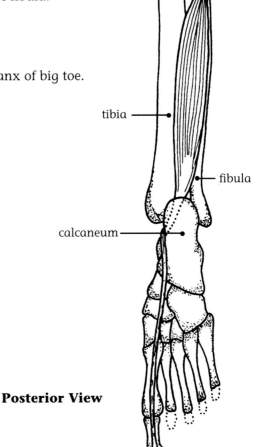

tibia

fibula

calcaneum

Posterior View

WATCH OUT!

The long tendon of this muscle is the weak area and is liable to become inflamed due to excess pressure or overuse.

Extensor Hallucis Longus

(Latin: **extendere** - to stretch, **hallux** - big toe).

BODY LANGUAGE OF WEAKNESS

Inability to extend big toe.

FINGER FIRST AID

Stretch and massage big toe and top side of foot.

Action

Extends big toe and assists in dorsiflexion of foot.

Origin

Middle half of the front surface of the fibula.

Insertion

Last phalanx of the big toe.

tibia

fibula

WATCH OUT!

The tendon is damaged by compression and by bruising if the toe is stepped on!

Hamstrings

(German: **hamme** - back of leg.
Latin: **stringere** - to draw
together).

'Knock knees', weakness on the
inside of the knee, or 'bow legs'
when the weakness is on the
outside of the knee.

FINGER FIRST AID

Rub origin and insertion of
muscle. Also press into belly of
muscle.

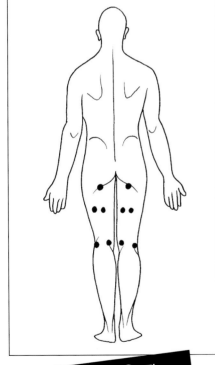

**Posterior
View**

*The hamstrings consist
of three muscles - two
medial (on the inside of
the thigh), called the
semitendinosus and
the semimembranosus
and one lateral (on the
outside of the thigh),
called the biceps
femoris.*

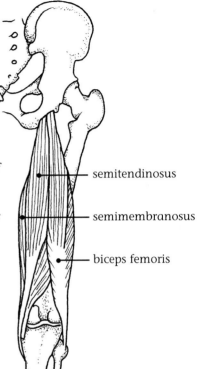

semitendinosus

semimembranosus

biceps femoris

Action	Flexes the knee, extends the thigh.
Origin	Ischial tuberosity (bottom part of the pelvis) and the lower back portion of the femur.
Insertion	Either side of the tibia, at the back.
Synergists	Gastrocnemius, gracilis, sartorius.
Alternative connections	Problems with these muscles may be associated with toxic conditions of the body involving the large intestine. Also from sacral and pelvic fixations. Vitamin E helps.

WATCH OUT!

These muscles are often injured when dancers do the
splits without proper warm-up. Also when kicking to the front.

Quadriceps

(Latin: **quad** - four, **caput** - head).

*The quadriceps are made up of four muscles. One, the **rectus femoris**, crosses both the hip and knee joint. The other three; **vastus medialis**, **vastus intermedius** and **vastus lateralis** act on the knee joint only.*

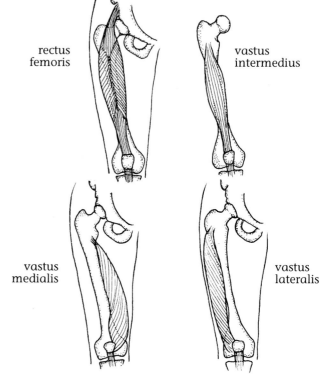

rectus femoris

vastus intermedius

vastus medialis

vastus lateralis

WATCH OUT!

Action	Extends the leg and flexes the thigh.
Origin	Rectus femoris: front point of the ilium. Vastus group; upper portion of the femur.
Insertion	The upper portion of the patella and via the patellar ligament into the tibia.
Synergists	Psoas, sartorius, tensor fascia lata.

Many problems with the knees can be traced back to faulty training techniques which have not taken into account the need to stretch and exercise all parts of the quadriceps. Often dancers suffer from an imbalance between the vastus medialis and the vastus lateralis. This leads to an uneven pull on the patella and is often the precursor to a condition called chondromalacia patella (excess wear on the articular surface between femur and patella).

Sartorius

(Latin: **sartor** - tailor, as in sitting cross-legged).

Weakness of this muscle can cause knee problems, especially on the inside of the knee (knock knees).

FINGER FIRST AID

Massage the whole muscle, paying special attention to the origin and insertion points

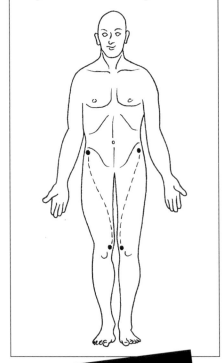

WATCH OUT!

Action

Flexes knee and hip, rotates the thigh laterally (turns outwards).

Origin

Front point of ilium.

Insertion

Medial surface of tibia.

Synergists

Quadriceps, hamstrings, gracilis.

Alternative connections

This muscle is very sensitive to adrenal exhaustion which often manifests as low blood sugar, low resistance to infections and asthma. Vitamin C can help.

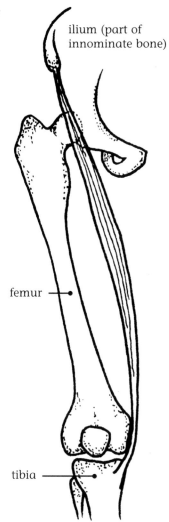

ilium (part of innominate bone)

femur

tibia

Anterior View

Turning out the leg puts great stress on the inside of the knee and often trouble here can be traced to a hypertonic (over-tense) sartorius.

Gracilis

(Latin: **gracilis** - slender).

Lack of pelvic stability, 'knock knee' problems.

FINGER FIRST AID

Origin and insertion massage, also pressure into the belly of the muscle.

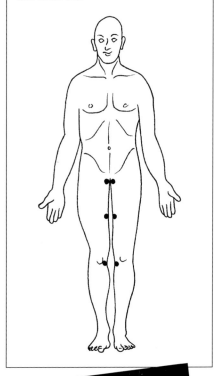

Action

Adducts thigh, flexes knee and hip and medially rotates the thigh and tibia (rotates them inwards).

Origin

Lower edge of pubic bone.

Insertion

Upper part of the inside of the tibia.

Synergists

Adductors, sartorius and hamstring.

pubic bone

femur

tibia

Anterior View

WATCH OUT!

Groin strains and low back problems involving sacroiliac strains are common. Turning out the legs leads to excess tension in this muscle which is then expected to stretch beyond its limits.

Tensor Fascia Lata

(Latin: **tendere** - to stretch, **fascia** - band, bandage, **lateralis** - side).

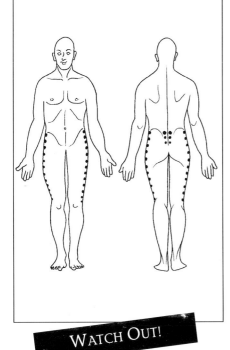

Action

Flexes, abducts and medially rotates the thigh (rotates it inwards). Also stabilises the outside of the knee.

Origin

Outer edge of the ilium, toward the front.

Insertion

Via the long fascia lata tendon to the outside top of the tibia.

Synergists

Gluteus medius and minimus.

Alternative connections

Linked with problems involving the large intestine such as constipation, colitis and diarrhoea. Increase water intake and natural sources of iron.

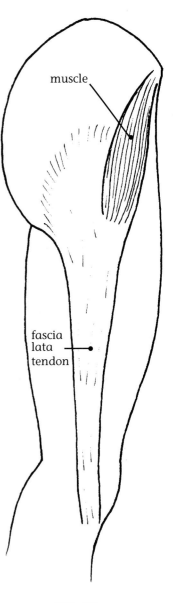

muscle

fascia lata tendon

Side View

Often becomes hypertonic (over-tense), causing lack of pelvic mobility and knee pain on the outside of the knee.

Adductors

(Latin: **ad** - to, **ducere** - to bring).

This group is actually four muscles: the pectineus adductor and the adductor brevis, longus and magnus.

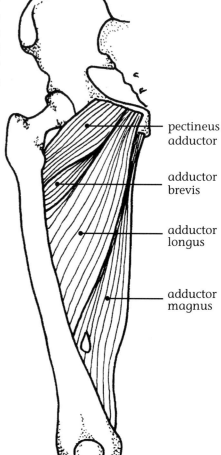

pectineus adductor

adductor brevis

adductor longus

adductor magnus

Action

Adduction, hip flexion and lateral rotation of the thigh.

Origin

Front part of pubic bone and lower part of hip bone (ischial tuberosity).

Insertion

Inside of the femur from hip to knee.

Synergists

Gracilis.

WATCH OUT!

Groin strains are common with these muscles. They become hypertonic through over-use and when stretched often tear.

Gluteus Medius/Minimus

(Greek: **gloutos** - rump. Latin: **medius** - middle, **minimus** - smallest).

Hips uneven, shoulders uneven. Difficulty keeping pelvis level when standing on one leg.

FINGER FIRST AID

Rub firmly front of body, above the pubic bone and above the thigh; back, inside the prominent knobs on the hip bones at the level of the 5th lumbar joint. Also origin and insertion technique.

WATCH OUT!

gluteus minimus

This lies under the gluteus medius.

Posterior View

gluteus medius

Action	Abducts thigh, medial rotators.
Origin	Outer surface of ilium.
Insertion	Top of femur to the side.
Synergists	Tensor fascia lata.

Excess tension or weakness in these muscles can lead to problems with the pelvis or knees due to compensation of other muscles.

Piriformis

(Greek: **pyramis** - pyramid shaped).

Difficulty turning the leg out.

FINGER FIRST AID

Rub firmly the top of pubic bone and above the thigh on the front of body, and inside the prominent knobs on the hip bones at the level of the 5th lumbar joint on the back. Also try deep pressure into the belly (a point between sacrum and femur, beneath the gluteus maximus) - you have to press quite hard, so be careful.

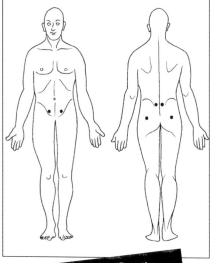

WATCH OUT!

Action

Rotates thigh laterally (turns it out). Abducts thigh when leg is flexed.

Origin

Front of sacrum.

Insertion

Top of femur.

Alternative connections

Problems with the piriformis often affect the sciatic nerve. This can cause pain down the back of the leg, numbness, tingling and sometimes bladder problems.

Posterior View

sacrum

femur

Anterior View

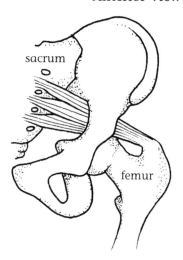

sacrum

femur

This muscle does most of the work when you turn out the leg.

This muscle usually becomes hypertonic (over-tense), which leads to a restriction of mobility in the hip. Pushing the turn-out without realising the root of the problem can often lead to injury. This is experienced as pain inside the hip or low back, or sciatica (pain down the back of the leg).

Gluteus Maximus

(Greek: **gloutos** - rump. Latin: **maximus** - biggest).

FINGER FIRST AID

Origin and insertion technique. Also massage firmly the vastus lateralis muscle down the outside of the thigh.

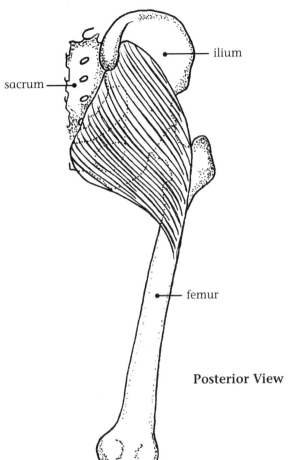

Posterior View

Action	Extends hip, laterally rotates high (assists turn-out).
Origin	Back of the ilium along the sacroiliac joint.
Insertion	Top back of the femur.
Synergists	Hamstrings.

WATCH OUT!

Low back problems due to excess lordosis (sway back). Difficulty maintaining straight spine when jumping.

Psoas/Iliacus (Iliopsoas)

(Greek: **psoas** - tenderloin. Latin: **ilium** - hip bone).

These two muscles will be considered as one.

Excess or diminished lumbar curve. Spine tilted away from the weak side.

These muscles are too deep, so use reflex points. Press deeply into the abdomen, one inch to the side and one inch above the navel. Also on the back, either side of the 12th thoracic/1st lumbar joints.

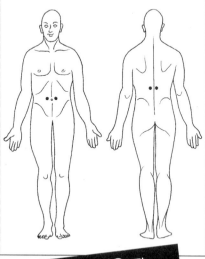

WATCH OUT!

Action

Flexes thigh, aids slightly in lateral rotation (turn-out).

Origin

Psoas: front surfaces of the transverse processes of the vertebrae from the 12th thoracic to the 5th lumbar joints.
Iliacus: the front inside of the ilium and sacrum.

Insertion

Inside top of the femur.

psoas

iliacus

Anterior View

Synergists
Adductors, rectus femoris.

Alternative connections   Nagging low back pain, kidney disturbances, low energy and foot difficulties can be associated with psoas problems. Drink water regularly. Vitamins A and E help.

This is the main hip flexor and low back stabiliser.
If these muscles go out of balance (usually by becoming hypertonic), then all kinds of low back and hip problems can develop.

Abdominals

(Latin: **abdomen** - belly)

BODY LANGUAGE OF WEAKNESS

Excess lumbar curvature (lordosis) and an inability to stabilise the lower back and pelvis when lifting one leg off the ground.

FINGER FIRST AID

Origin and insertion technique. Also watch the lower part of the rectus abdominals for weakness. If the pelvis is tilted forward when standing, or if there is an excessive hollow in the back when lying down, suspect a weakness here.

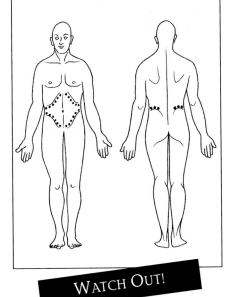

WATCH OUT!

Action	**Transverse**: constricts abdominal contents, assists in forcing air out of lungs.

Transverse: constricts abdominal contents, assists in forcing air out of lungs.
Rectus: gives anterior support to lumbar spine, holds rib cage and pubis together.
Internal/external obliques: flex, rotate and side-bend trunk.

There are four main divisions of abdominal muscles

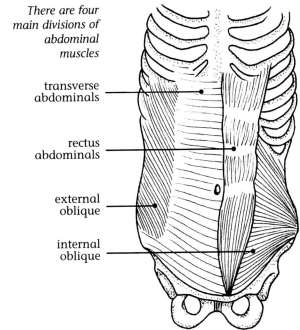

transverse abdominals

rectus abdominals

external oblique

internal oblique

Origin   Ribs.

Insertion   Upper edges of ilium and pubic bones.

Synergists   Iliopsoas.

Alternative connections   Digestive problems, particularly those involving the small intestine, are associated with these muscles. Good abdominal tone supports the internal organs, Vitamin E helps.

The lower lumbar joints are most at risk when the abdominals and the iliopsoas muscles have to work together in order to keep the spine stable. One without the other creates an imbalance which eventually will lead to injury.

Bibliography

Anderson, Bob; **Stretching**, Shelter Publications, Bolinas, California, 1987.

Anthony and Thibodeau; **Textbook of Anatomy and Physiology**, The C. V. Mosby Company, St. Louis, Toronto, London, 1983.

Despard, L. L.; **Textbook of Massage**, Oxford University Press, London, 1914.

Hoppenfield, Stanley; **Physical Examination of the Spine and Extremities**, Appleton-Century-Crofts, New York, 1976.

Houston, F. M. and D. C.; **The Healing Benefits of Acupuncture**, Keats Publishing, New Canaan, Connecticut, 1970.

Hurley and Sanders; **Aquarian Age Bio-Engineering**, Los Angeles Health Research, 1970.

Irwin, Yukiko; **Shiatzu**, Routledge & Kegan Paul, London, 1977.

Kapandji, I. A.; **The Physiology of the Joints**, Churchill Livingstone, Edinburgh, London, New York, 1974.

Kapit and Elson; **The Anatomy Colouring Book**, Harper and Row, New York, San Francisco, 1977.

Kennedy, Pat; **The Moving Body**, Faber and Faber, London, 1979.

Kushi, Michio; **How to see your Health: Handbook of Oriental Diagnosis**, Japan Publications Inc., Tokyo, 1975.

McNaught and Callander; **Nurses' Illustrated Physiology**, Churchill Livingstone, Edinburgh, London, New York, 1975.

Pearce, Evelyn; **Anatomy and Physiology for Nurses**, Faber and Faber, London, 1981.

Rowlett, H.; **Basic Anatomy and Physiology**, John Murray, London, 1979.

Sparger, Celia; **Ballet Physique**, Adam and Charles Black, London, 1958.

Thie, John; **Touch for Health**, DeVorss and Company, Marina del Rey, California, 1979.

Topping, Wayne; **Stress Release**, Topping International Institute, Bellingham, 1985.

Walther, David; **Applied Kinesiology**, Systems DC, Pueblo, Colorado, 1981.

Wheeler, C. M.; **Illustrated Human Biology**, Edward Arnold, London, 1978.

Wirhed, Rolf; **Athletic Ability and the Anatomy of Motion**, Wolfe Medical Publications, London, 1984.

Index

Index (cont.)

Q

Quadratus Lumborum, 9, 12
Quadriceps, 8, 36

R

Radius, 6, 7
Rhomboid, 9, 17
Ribs, 6
Rolling inwards of the foot, 30, 31
Rotation, description of the term, 5

S

Sacral fixation, 35
Sacrospinalis, 9, 11
Sacrum, 6, 7
Sartorius, 8, 37
Scapula, 7
    loss of mobility, 18
    winging, 19
Sciatica, 42
Serratus Anterior, 8, 19
Shin splints, 30
Shoulder problems, 16, 17, 18, 19,
    20, 23, 24, 25, 27, 41
Side bending, related injury, 12, 44
Sinus, associated problems, 10
Skeleton, 6, 7
Splits, associated muscles, 35
Soleus, 9, 29
Sternum, 6
Sternocleidomastoid, 8, 10
Stress, 21, 37
Subscapularis, 8, 25
Sugar metabolism, related
    muscles, 13, 20
Synergist, description of term, 4

T

Tarsal bones, 6, 7
Tennis elbow, 15
Teres Major, 9, 24
Teres Minor, 9, 26
Tensor Fascia Lata, 8, 39
Thoracic vertebrae, 7
Tibia, 6, 7
Turn out, 40, 42
Triceps, 9, 13
Triceps tendon, 13

U

Ulna, 6, 7

V

Vitamins, associated muscles
    Vitamin A, 11, 13, 16, 17, 20,
    25, 44
    Vitamin B, 10, 16, 21
    Vitamin C, 11, 16, 19, 22, 28,
    29, 37
    Vitamin E, 25, 30, 35, 44, 45

W

Waking up a weak muscle (see
    origin and insertion
    technique), 5
Watch Out, 4
Whiplash, 10
Wrist extensors, 8, 15
Wrist flexors, 8, 15
Wrist problems, 26

The main building of the Institute headquarters, near Honesdale, Pennsylvania.

The Himalayan Institute

FOUNDED IN 1971 by Swami Rama, the Himalayan Institute has been dedicated to helping people grow physically, mentally, and spiritually by combining the best knowledge of both the East and the West.

Our international headquarters is located on a beautiful 400-acre campus in the rolling hills of the Pocono Mountains of northeastern Pennsylvania. The atmosphere here is one to foster growth, increased inner awareness, and calm. Our grounds provide a wonderfully peaceful and healthy setting for our seminars and extended programs. Students from around the world join us here to attend programs in such diverse areas as hatha yoga, meditation, stress reduction, Ayurveda, nutrition, Eastern philosophy, psychology, and other subjects. Whether the programs are for weekend meditation retreats, week-long seminars on spirituality, months-long residential programs, or holistic health services, the attempt here is to provide an environment of gentle inner progress. We invite you to join with us in the ongoing process of personal growth and development.

The Institute is a nonprofit organization. Your membership in the Institute helps to support its programs. Please call or write for information on becoming a member.

Institute Programs, Services, and Facilities

Institute programs share an emphasis on conscious holistic living and personal self-development, including:

Special weekend or extended seminars to teach skills and techniques for increasing your ability to be healthy and enjoy life

Meditation retreats and advanced meditation and
philosophical instruction

Vegetarian cooking and nutritional training

Hatha yoga and exercise workshops

Residential programs for self-development

Holistic health services and Ayurvedic Rejuvenation
Programs through the Institute's Center for Health
and Healing.

A Quarterly Guide to Programs and Other Offerings is free within
the USA. To request a copy, or for further information, call
800-822-4547 or 570-253-5551, fax 570-253-9078, email
bqinfo@himalayaninstitute.org, write the Himalayan Institute,
RR 1 Box 1127, Honesdale, PA 18431-9706 USA, or visit our Web
site at www.himalayaninstitute.org.

The Himalayan Institute Press

THE HIMALAYAN INSTITUTE PRESS has long been regarded as
"The Resource for Holistic Living." We publish dozens of titles, as
well as audio and video tapes, that offer practical methods for
living harmoniously and achieving inner balance. Our
approach addresses the whole person—body, mind, and
spirit—integrating the latest scientific knowledge with ancient
healing and self-development techniques.

As such, we offer a wide array of titles on physical and
psychological health and well-being, spiritual growth through
meditation and other yogic practices, as well as translations of
yogic scriptures.

Our sidelines include the Japa Kit for meditation practice,
the Neti™ Pot, the ideal tool for sinus and allergy sufferers, and
The Breath Pillow,™ a unique tool for learning health-supportive
diaphragmatic breathing.

Subscriptions are available to a bimonthly magazine, *Yoga
International*, which offers thought-provoking articles on all
aspects of meditation and yoga, including yoga's sister science,
Ayurveda.

For a free catalog call 800-822-4547 or 570-253-5551, email
hibooks@himalayaninstitute.org, fax 570-253-6360, write the
Himalayan Institute Press, RR 1, Box 1129, Honesdale, PA 18431-
9709, USA, or visit our Web site at www.himalayaninstitute.org.